The Handbook for

The Cardiovascular System

Isabella Woodbridge

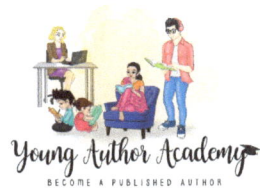

"The Handbook for The Cardiovascular System"

published through Young Author Academy Publishing.

ISBN: 9798869579669

Printed by Amazon Direct Publishing.

INTRODUCTION

Whether characterised into a symmetrical shape representing love or labelled with immense detail, the heart is an incredible organ that has been developed naturally with such a system that is so advanced and yet quite simple.

The Cardiovascular System is a system including the heart and blood vessels and is the main component of what keeps us alive. Over the years, we have discovered more and more about the system and what can cause it to fail such as heart attacks, arrhythmia and high blood pressure (hypertension).

TO THE
CARDIOVASCULAR SYSTEM

The heart is an extremely important organ and the majority of lifestyles people warn about mainly affect the heart, which cannot only exert symptoms but can cause symptoms in other organs and tissues in the body.

In this book, we will talk about the incredible feats of the heart, how it works and where it can go wrong when it fails or starts to fail.

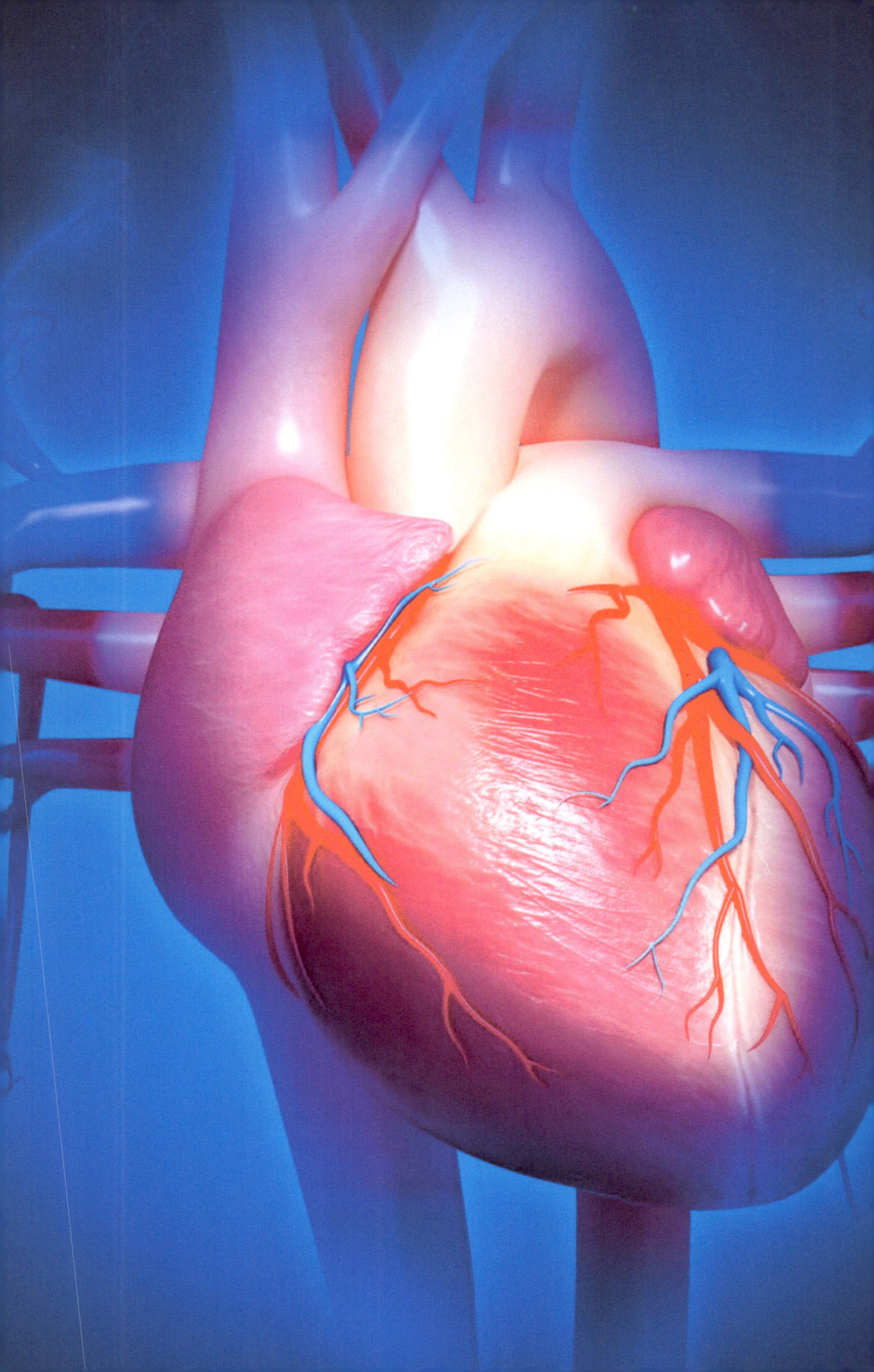

THE HEART,

THE ANATOMY

THE HEART

What is in the heart? The heart contains many intricate parts with specific functions that keep us alive. These are listed below:

- *Right Atrium*: Takes in deoxygenated (without oxygen) blood from the body through the **superior** and **inferior vena cava** and contracts to pump the blood into the right ventricle through the **tricuspid valve**.
- *Tricuspid valve*: A three-cusped valve between the right atrium and right ventricle.
- *Septum*: To separate deoxygenated and oxygenated blood.
- *Superior and inferior vena cava*: Superior vena cava takes in deoxygenated blood from the top part of the body while the inferior vena cava takes in deoxygenated blood from the bottom part of the body.
- *Right Ventricle*: Pumps deoxygenated blood through the **pulmonary valve** and **pulmonary artery** towards the lungs to get oxygenated through gas exchange.
- *Pulmonary valve*: A valve between the right ventricle and **pulmonary artery**.
- *Left Atrium*: Takes in oxygenated blood through the **pulmonary vein** from the lungs and pumps it through the **mitral valve** into the **left ventricle**.
- *Left Ventricle*: Takes in oxygenated blood through the **pulmonary vein** from the lungs and pumps it through the **mitral valve** into
- *Mitral valve*: A valve between the left atrium and left ventricle.

DIAGRAM

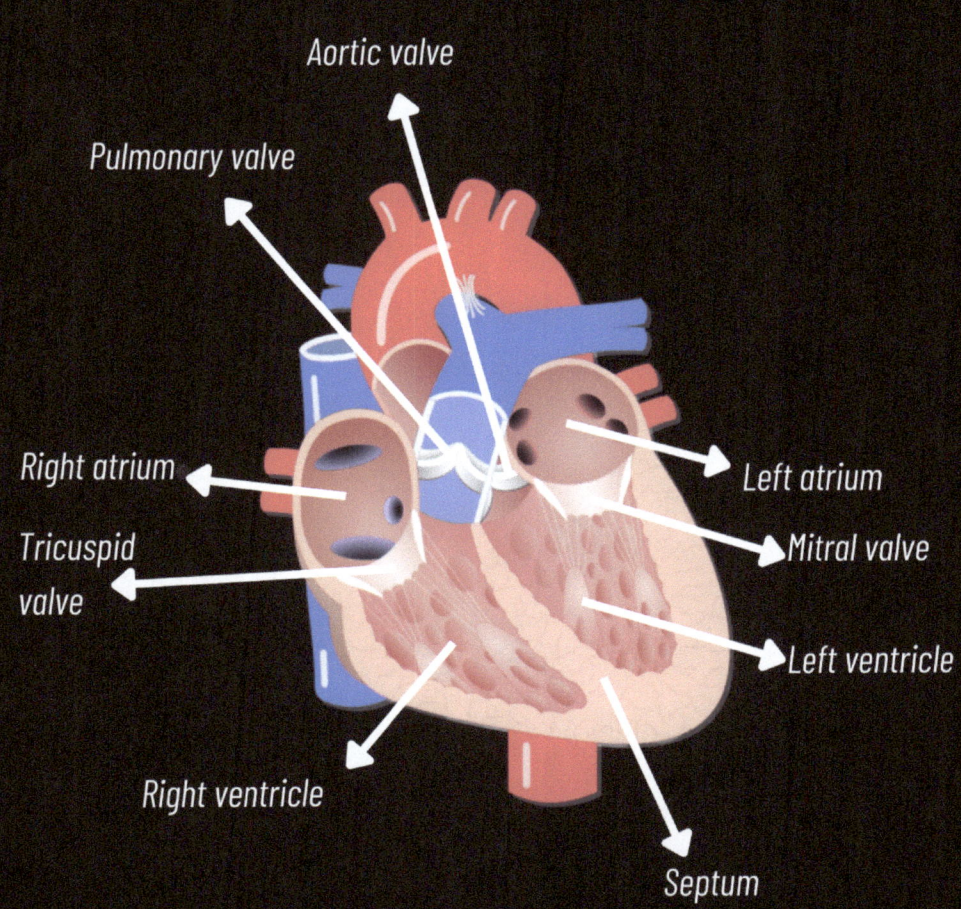

Aortic valve

Pulmonary valve

Right atrium

Tricuspid valve

Left atrium

Mitral valve

Right ventricle

Left ventricle

Septum

THE HEART

What is in the heart?

The heart contains many intricate parts with specific functions that keep us alive. These are listed below:

- *Aorta:* An artery that carries oxygenated blood from the left ventricle to the body.
- *Pulmonary artery*: An artery that takes deoxygenated blood from the right ventricle towards the lungs to get oxygenated.
- *Pulmonary vein*: A vein that takes oxygenated blood from the lungs into the left atrium.
- *Superior and inferior vena cava*: Superior vena cava takes in deoxygenated blood from the top part of the body while the inferior vena cava takes in deoxygenated blood from the bottom part of the body.
- *Right Coronary Artery:* An artery that supplies blood, and therefore oxygen, to the right atrium and ventricle, sinoatrial and atrioventricular node, tissues specialised to regulate the heart's contractions.
- *Circumflex Coronary Artery*: An artery that supplies blood, and therefore oxygen, to the left atrium and ventricle.
- *Left Anterior Descending Coronary Artery*: An artery that supplies blood, and therefore oxygen, to the right and left ventricle and the septum between ventricles.

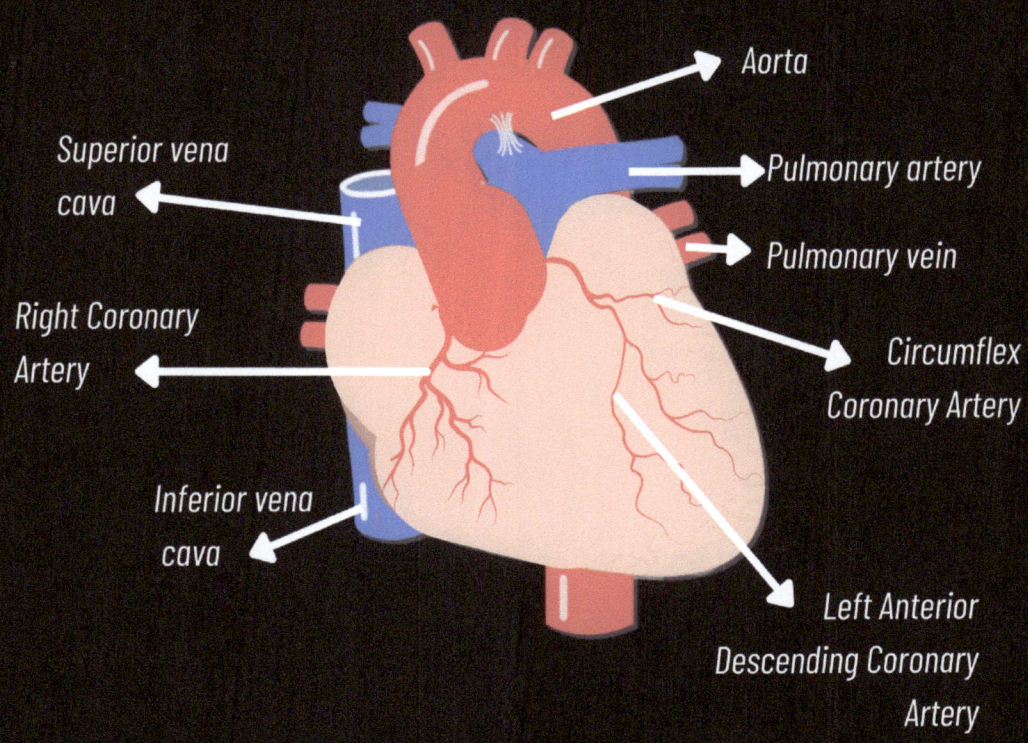

Aorta

Superior vena cava

Pulmonary artery

Pulmonary vein

Right Coronary Artery

Circumflex Coronary Artery

Inferior vena cava

Left Anterior Descending Coronary Artery

RESPIRATION

How are the muscles in the heart {known as the Myocardium} provided with energy to contract? Well, it is yielded through the process, Aerobic Respiration. This process takes in glucose, a simple sugar, from food and oxygen that we breathe in to provide us with energy, this produces carbon dioxide and water as byproducts, which we then rid of via exhalation. This is shown through the formulaic equation:

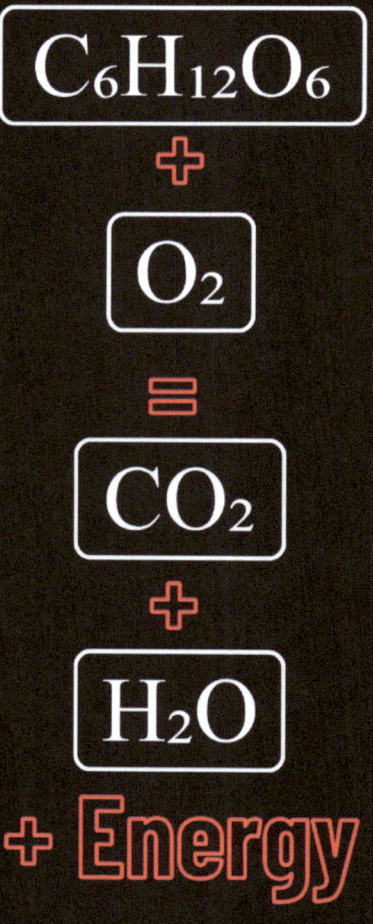

$$C_6H_{12}O_6 + O_2 = CO_2 + H_2O + Energy$$

ANAEROBIC RESPIRATION

The formula shown on the opposite page shows aerobic respiration, or respiration that uses oxygen. However, in cases of little oxygen, anaerobic respiration is used for a few moments. Instead of using glucose and oxygen, only glucose is used, yielding energy and producing lactic acid as a byproduct, which can cause cramps. In order to break down this lactic acid to avoid toxicity and damage, oxygen is needed to break it down into carbon dioxide and water. This is known as the oxygen debt which, once is cleared, will cause the cramps to disappear.

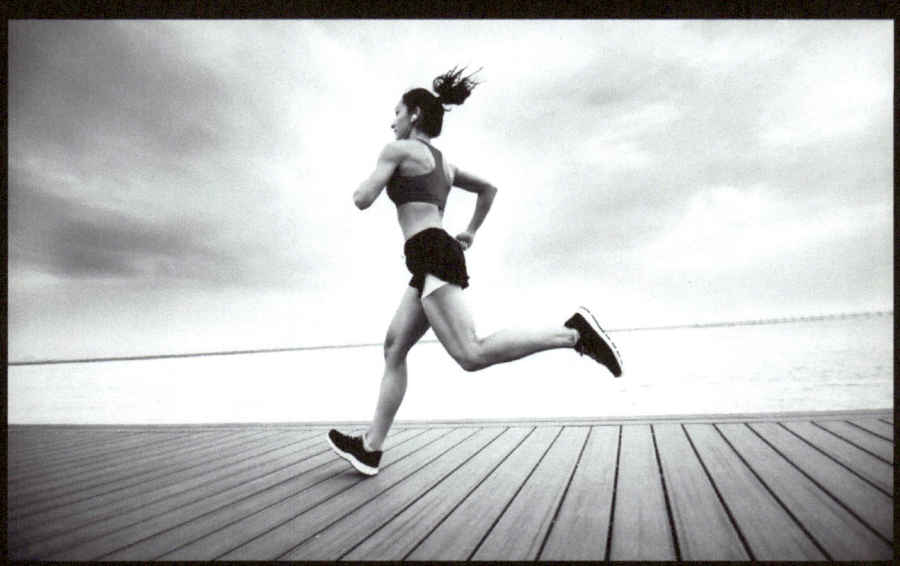

THE ROLE

As mentioned in the page prior, blood becomes oxygenated when it travels to the lungs, but how exactly?

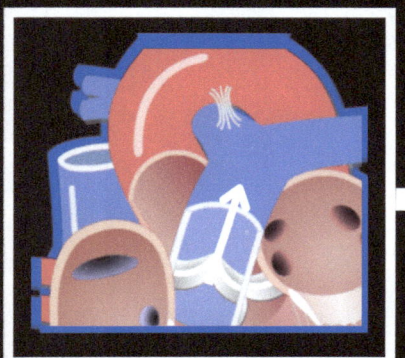

Deoxygenated blood is pumped through the pulmonary artery from the right ventricle.

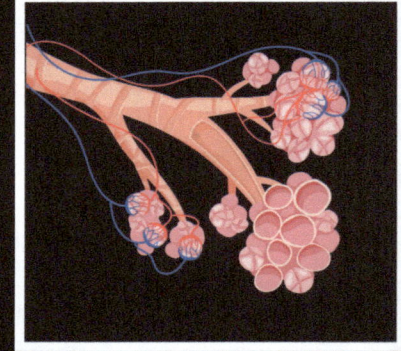

The pulmonary artery branches off into smaller blood vessels, eventually capillaries that line the alveoli (small air pockets in your lungs)

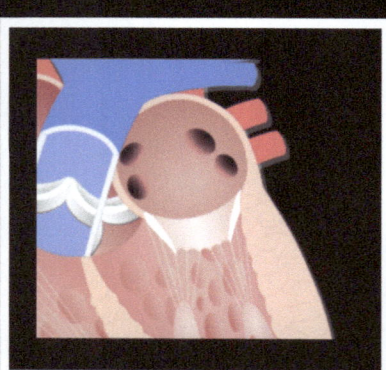

The now-oxygenated blood is transported back to the left atrium.

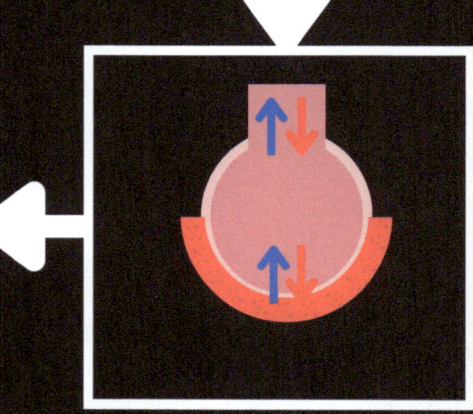

Oxygen is diffused to the red blood cells. Carbon Dioxide is diffused to the alveolus from the RBC.

OF OXYGEN

GAS EXCHANGE

Gas exchange between alveoli and blood vessels utilises a process known as diffusion, where particles in an area of high concentration move towards an area of low concentration.

In this case, alveoli are constantly expelling carbon dioxide and taking in oxygen, which means the alveolus has a high concentration of oxygen and a low concentration of carbon dioxide. So when deoxygenated red blood cells pass, the oxygen molecules diffuse from the alveoli (high concentration) to the red blood cells (low concentration) and the carbon dioxide molecules diffuse from the red blood cells (high concentration) to the alveoli. When the person exhales and then inhales, it re-establishes the high concentration of oxygen and low concentration of carbon dioxide in the alveoli.

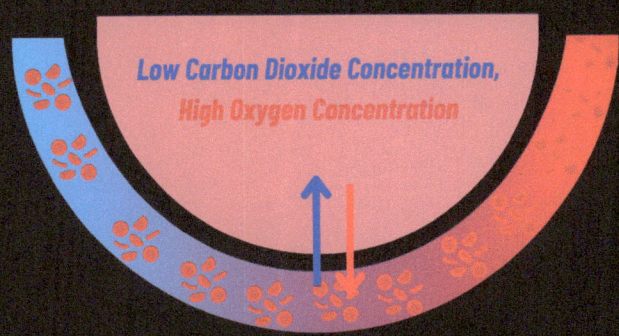

Low Carbon Dioxide Concentration, High Oxygen Concentration

Low Oxygen Concentration, High Carbon Dioxide Concentration

TYPES OF

RED BLOOD CELLS

Red blood cells are a type of blood cell that transports nutrients and gases. It most importantly transports oxygen binded to a protein known as haemoglobin to tissues in order for them to perform anaerobic respiration.

Red blood cells are adapted to not have a nucleus in order to have a larger surface area to absorb more oxygen.

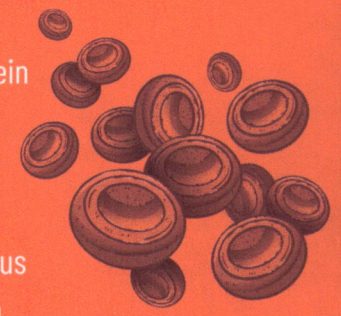

WHITE BLOOD CELLS

White blood cells are a type of blood cell that is focused on preventing and stopping pathogens from damaging the body. One type of white blood cells are lymphocytes which can come in the form of T-Cells, which destroy cells already infected by pathogens, and B-cells, which produce antibodies in order to attack invading pathogens.

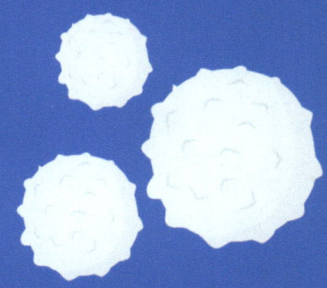

BLOOD CELLS

PLATELETS

Platelets are cell fragments that are used to stop any bleeds from blood vessels.

The body sends signals to trigger the response of platelets to the damaged area and clot the area. However in some cases, such as the damage of plaque buildup, platelets can clot in unwanted areas and cause a blockage of blood flow and infarction (tissue death due to lack of blood flow and therefore oxygen).

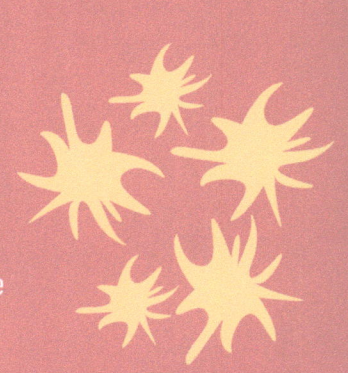

How do antibodies defend against pathogens?

Antibodies can signal pathogens by binding to proteins surrounding the pathogen cell known as antigens, triggering the response of other immune cells.

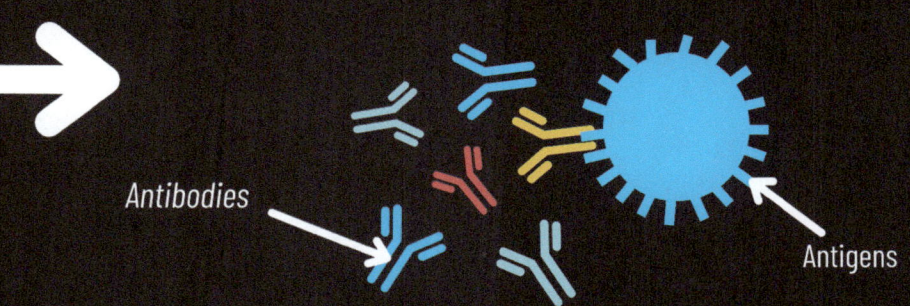

Antibodies

Antigens

ARTERIES &

There are three types of blood vessel: arteries, veins and capillaries. Each of these have a different function in the body and are adapted in order to support these functions.

Arteries: *Arteries contain blood of a very high blood pressure and therefore require a thick outer layer, and a thick elastic fibre and muscle layer. This leads to a small lumen, the area in the middle.*

Veins: *Veins, unlike arteries, contain blood at low pressure. This means that they have a thin outer layer and muscle/elastic fibre layer. However, veins have valves that stop the blood from travelling backwards through the blood vessel.*

Capillaries: *Capillaries have a very thin outer layer, only about one-cell thick. This it to allow the diffusion of substances across the surface.*

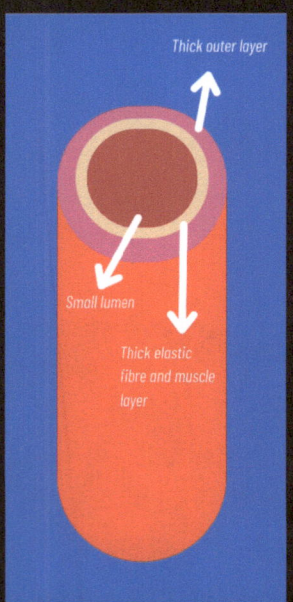

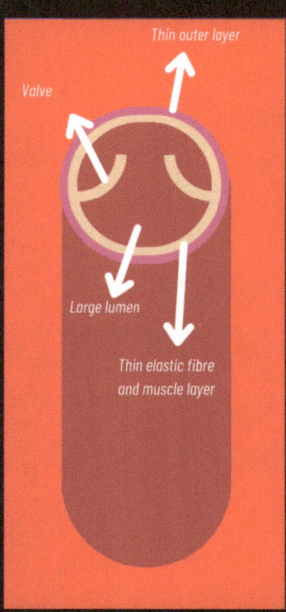

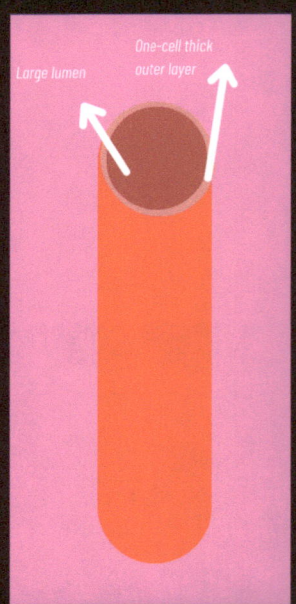

BLOOD PRESSURE

Blood pressure is the measure of pressure of blood against the walls of the arteries. Blood pressure is displayed as two numbers: the top is the systolic blood pressure, which is the blood pressure during heart contractions, and the bottom number is diastolic blood pressure, the blood pressure between contractions when the heart is at rest.

VEINS

Healthy blood pressure is where the systolic blood pressure is less than 120 and the diastolic blood pressure is less than 80. Anything significantly higher in both these categories is known as hypertension (high blood pressure).

	Systolic		Diastolic
HEALTHY BP	LESS THAN 120	and	LESS THAN 80
ELEVATED	120-129	and	LESS THAN 80
HYPERTENSION STAGE I	130-139	or	80-89
HYPERTENSION STAGE II	140 or HIGHER	or	90 or HIGHER
HYPERTENSIVE CRISIS	180 or HIGHER	and /or	120 or HIGHER

CONDITIONS

While our heart is an interesting and complex organ, there is still a lot that can go wrong.

MYOCARDIAL INFARCTION/HEART ATTACK

In a heart attack, technically known as a **myocardial infarction**, an artery known as the **coronary artery** becomes blocked due to a condition known as atherosclerosis (shown below), causing the myocardium around the heart to lack in oxygen and therefore lack in energy via respiration.

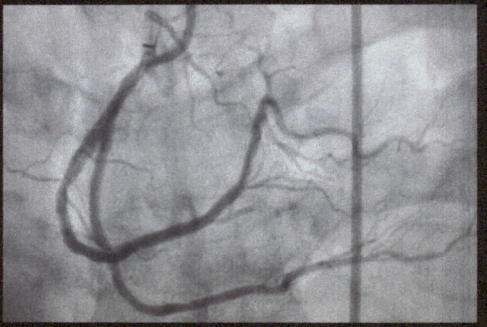

ATHEROSCLEROSIS

Atherosclerosis is a condition where an artery becomes blocked due to plaque build up (as shown to the right). This can become worse if the plaque breaks as it can trigger a response where platelets attempt to fix the gap by attaching to the plaque, causing further blockage.

When this occurs in the coronary artery, the main artery that supplies blood (and subsequently oxygen) to the myocardium, which is the muscle that contracts in order to move blood, the heart's myocardium does not receive enough oxygen for aerobic respiration and therefore not enough energy to contract. This is known as a myocardial infarction or a heart attack (as shown above).

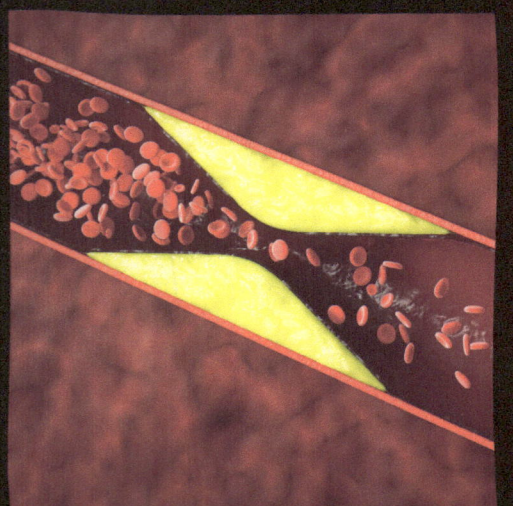

THROMBUS AND EMBOLUS

A **thrombus** is a clotted mass of blood that forms in a blood vessel, causing a blockage and therefore can cause a lack of blood flow to certain tissues causing inflammation/swelling, red and darkened skin and noticeable veins.

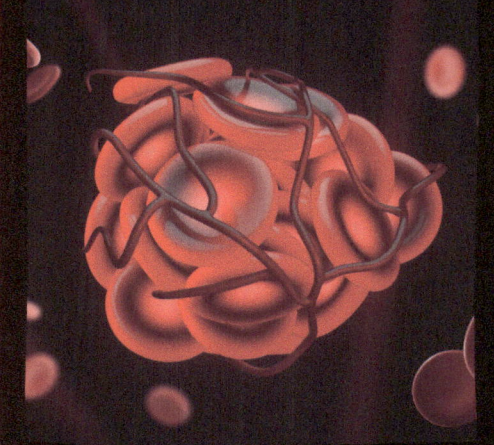

If a thrombus becomes loose and begins to travel through the bloodstream, it becomes an **embolus**. This means that it is a clot that will continue to move until it reaches an artery too narrow to move through the block the artery, causing an infarction. An example of a thrombus is a DVT (Deep-Vein Thrombosis) which can be caused by inactivity in the leg such as sitting for too long, combined with a family history of blood clots. However, this can become life-threatening in the case of a pulmonary embolism, where an embolus becomes lodged in the pulmonary arteries, causing a lack of blood flow to the lungs and symptoms like chest pain and severe difficulty breathing.

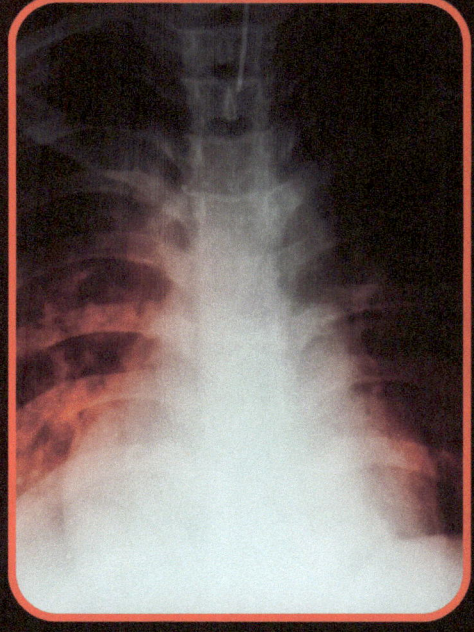

ARRYTHMIA

An arrhythmia is an irregularity of heart rate or rhythm. This can come in the form of bradycardia, where the heart rate is too slow, and tachycardia, where the heart rate is too fast.

It is mainly caused by irregular and chaotic signals that incorrectly contract the heart and cause an irregular rhythm.

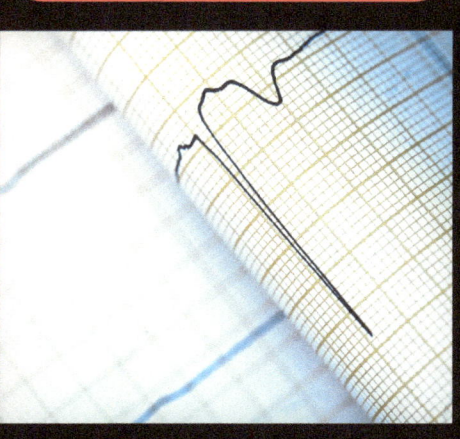

ANGINA PECTORIS

Chest pain caused by lack of blood flow towards the muscles in the heart (myocardium).

This is commonly caused by CAD, or cornary artery disease, shown on the opposite page.

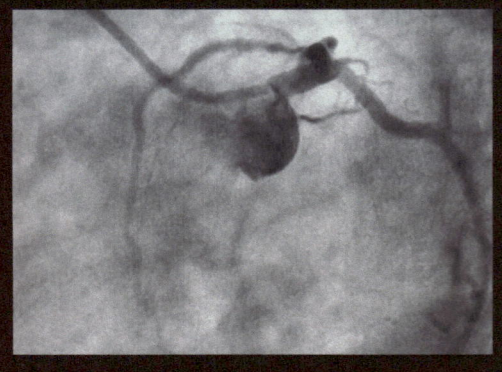

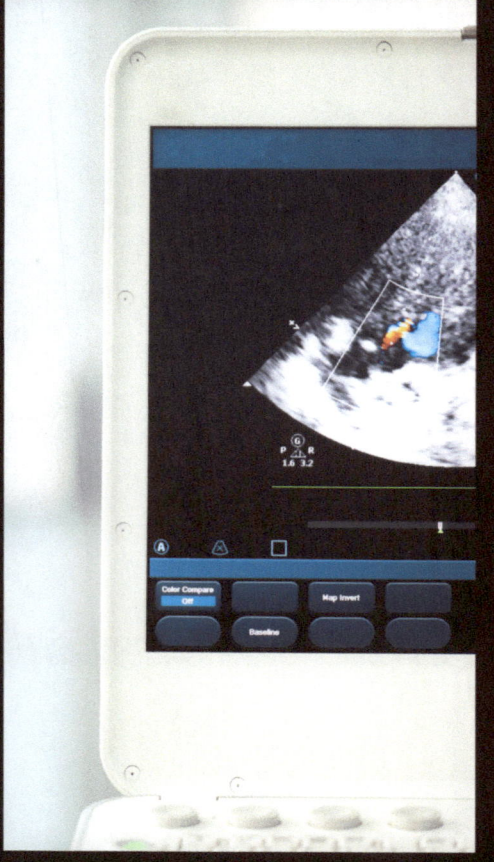

VALVE PROLAPSE AND REGURGITATION

In valve prolapse, one of the heart valves (tricuspid, mitral, aortic or pulmonary) are not as strong and are a lot more free-flowing. This can cause mild leaks backwards through the chambers.

When valve prolapse becomes much more severe in the form of valve regurgitation, more blood is flowing backwards which means that not enough blood is reaching important tissues.

Valve prolapse and regurgitation can be treated by performing a surgery known as annuloplasty, where a ring is secured around the valve to make it more stiff and strong.

The opposing condition is valve stenosis, where the valve tissue is too stiff and does not allow enough movement to move blood.

CORONARY ARTERY DISEASE

As shown on the previous pages, atherosclerosis forms from plaque buildup causing a clot or lack of blood flow. When this specifically occurs in the coronary artery, the artery supplying blood to the myocardium, it is known as coronary artery disease.

This condition can be treated through a surgery known as coronary angioplasty and stent placement, where a small metal mesh is placed to expand the artery, or coronary artery bypass graft (CABG), where a blood vessel from another area is placed where the coronary artery is to restructure around the clot.

STROKE

Strokes are caused by blood clots in the blood vessels supplying blood to the brain.

Depending on where the brain is affected, the symptoms can vary, however the main symptoms include: difficulty with speech (aphasia), weakness on one side of the body, lack of coordination and balance, dizziness and/or headache.

Strokes are usually treated by mechanical embolectomy, where the surgeon removes the buildup of plaque in the blood vessel affected.

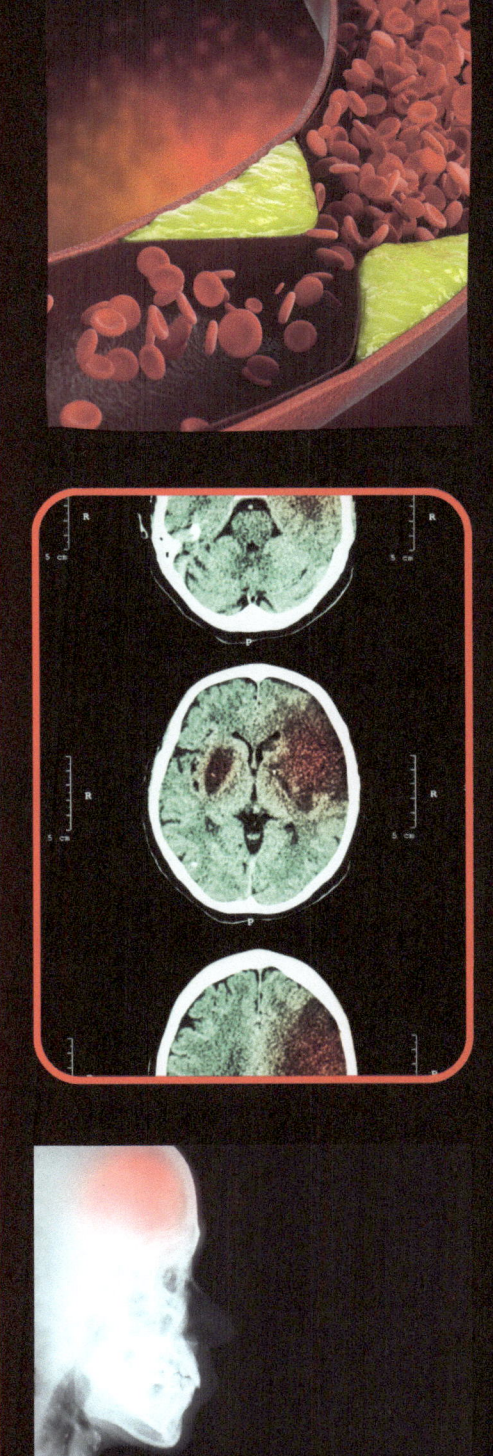

See the Other Titles in the Series:

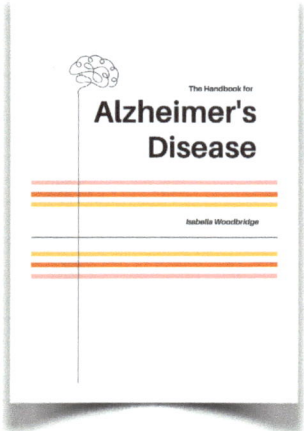

The Handbook for
Alzheimer's Disease